INTERMITTENT FASTING for Women

Over 60

"Unlocking Health, Energy, and Longevity with Tailored Fasting Strategies for the Wise and Wonderful women"

By

Linda A. Ivey

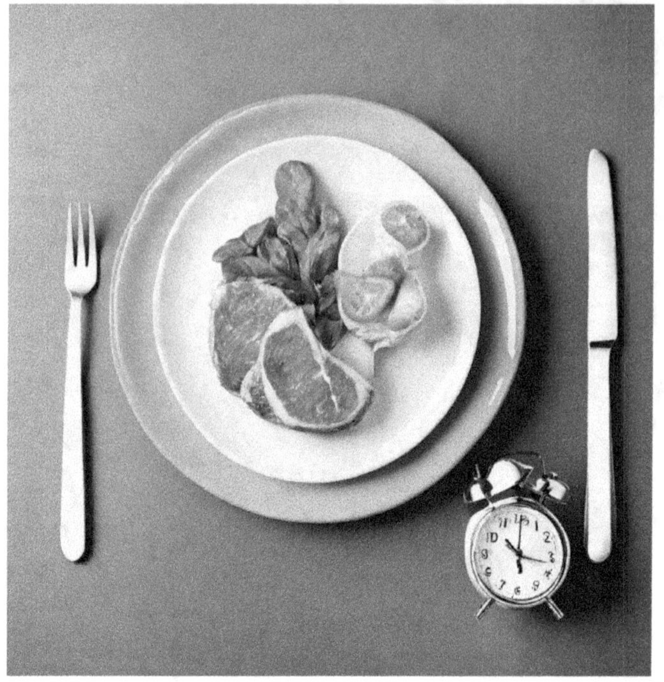

THANK YOU FOR CHOOSING US.

We Appreciate Your Kind Support And We Hope You Got Something Out Of It.

If You Enjoy This Book, It Will Be Great To Leave a Review On Amazon . It Means a Lot To Us.

Copyright ©y by Linda A. Ivey 2023.

Contents

Introduction

In the tapestry of life, wellness is a thread woven with the choices we make—choices that become increasingly vital as we embrace the wisdom and grace that come with age. For women over 60, the journey towards health is an ongoing adventure, and one approach that has captured the spotlight for its potential benefits is intermittent fasting.

As we navigate the realms of health and aging, this guide unfolds as a compass, directing attention to the profound impact that intermittent fasting can have on the well-being of women in their sixth decade and beyond. It is not just a diet but a lifestyle—a rhythmic dance with time that holds the promise of enhanced energy, vitality, and longevity.

Chapter by chapter, we will delve into the science behind intermittent fasting, explore its tailored benefits for women over 60, and equip ourselves with the knowledge needed to embark on this transformative journey. From understanding the crucial role of nutrient-rich foods to discovering the power of fasting-friendly ingredients, this guide sets the stage for a holistic and personalized approach to health.

But knowledge alone is not enough; practicality is the linchpin of sustainable change. Thus, we present a curated collection of delectable recipes designed to nourish the body during various fasting windows. From invigorating breakfasts to hearty dinners and guilt-free desserts, these recipes marry the principles of intermittent fasting with culinary delight, proving that healthful eating need not sacrifice flavor.

As we embark on this expedition together, let us embrace the beauty of self-care and celebrate the strength that comes from within. This guide is more than words on paper—it is an invitation to savor the richness of life through mindful choices, embracing the potential of intermittent fasting to unlock the door to a healthier, more vibrant you. Welcome to a journey of wellness tailor-made for the wise and wonderful women over 60.

Chapter 1

Embracing Intermittent Fasting

- ## The Science Behind Fasting

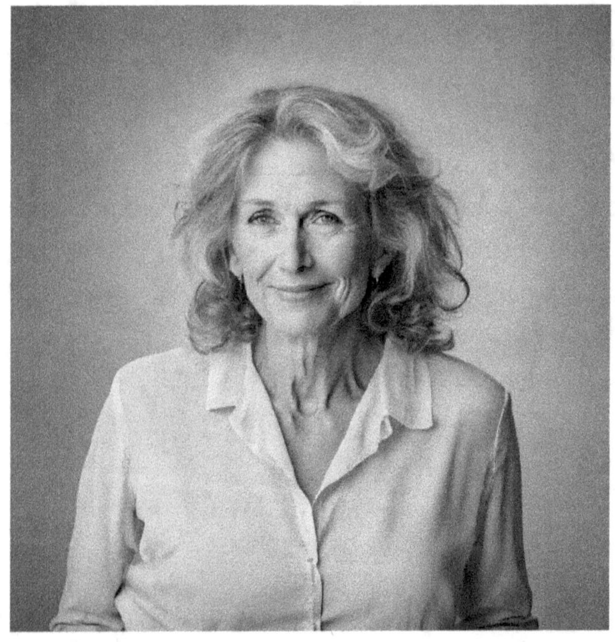

In recent years, fasting—an age-old habit with origins in many different cultural and spiritual traditions—has drawn significant scientific attention. Determining the scientific foundations that elevate intermittent fasting beyond a passing fad is crucial as we delve further into its nuances.

Fasting's Physiology

We explore the physiological changes that take place in the body when fasting in this section. We learn the processes that distinguish fasting as a metabolic transition that affects how our bodies make and use energy, from the depletion of glycogen reserves to the onset of ketosis.

Fasting and Hormones

Hormones are key to the complex dance of changes brought about by fasting. The effects of fasting on growth hormone, insulin, and other important endocrine system components are examined in this part. It is possible to get insight into how fasting may support weight control, metabolic health, and even lifespan by comprehending these hormonal changes.

Autophagy inside Cells

Autophagy, an internal recycling mechanism that gets rid of damaged cell components, is a phenomena that is becoming more and more well-known in the field of fasting study. We investigate how fasting stimulates autophagy, which may help cells regenerate and become more resistant to age-related illnesses.

Brain Health and Cognitive Advantages

Fasting has been connected to enhanced brain health and cognitive advantages in addition to its physical impacts. The neurological underpinnings of fasting are explored in this section, along with its potential benefits for improving mental health in general, preventing neurodegenerative illnesses, and improving cognitive performance.

Creating Customised Fasting for Women Abroad

The demands of women over 60 should be given particular care, even if the science of fasting is universal. This article explores how women's experiences with fasting may be impacted by the physiological changes that come with ageing, providing information on how to tailor and optimise for this particular group.

Equipped with a fundamental comprehension of the science behind fasting, we open the door for a more deliberate and knowledgeable investigation of intermittent fasting catered to the particular requirements of women beyond 60.

• Benefits for Women Over 60

It is important to understand the many advantages of intermittent fasting as it relates to the particular requirements and experiences of women who are approaching or have reached their sixth decade of life. In this chapter, we shed light on the transformational benefits of intermittent fasting, which promote a well-rounded approach to health.

• Balance of Hormones

Hormonal changes are a common side effect of ageing for women over 60. This section examines the possible benefits of intermittent fasting on hormonal balance, including the potential relief of menopausal symptoms and the enhancement of general reproductive health.

- **Mastery of Metabolism**

Age-related changes in metabolism make it more important than ever to maintain a healthy weight and metabolic function. Discover the potential benefits of intermittent fasting as a metabolic ally that may enhance metabolic resistance against ageing and help with weight control.

- **Clarity of Thought**

A key component of wellbeing is cognitive health, particularly for women managing the complex terrain of ageing. Learn how the neuroprotective benefits of intermittent fasting might improve cognitive performance and perhaps lower the risk of age-related cognitive decline.

- **Vitality of the Heart**

Heart health is very important, especially as people become older. The possible cardiovascular advantages of intermittent fasting are examined in this section, including how it may lower the risk of cardiovascular illnesses in women over 60, improve cholesterol profiles, and control blood pressure.

- ## **Understanding Longevity**

Everyone wants to age gracefully, and this article looks at the fascinating connection between lifespan and intermittent fasting. Discover the scientific data indicating that intermittent fasting may lead to a longer and healthier life, promising women over 60 years of age to live longer and more vibrant lives.

- ## **Bone Health and Absorption of Nutrients**

It becomes more and more important to keep your bones strong and healthy as you age. Examine the connection between bone health and intermittent fasting, and how it could affect the body's ability to absorb minerals that are vital for strong and resilient bones, such as calcium and vitamin D.

- ## **Increasing the Resilience of Cells**

Cellular resilience becomes more important as the body matures to counteract the consequences of inflammation and oxidative stress. Examine the ways in which intermittent fasting might stimulate processes for cellular repair, hence mitigating the risk of age-related illnesses and improving the general cellular health of women who are over 60.

- **Enhanced Sensitivity to Insulin**

As people age, their insulin sensitivity tends to decrease, which increases their risk of type 2 diabetes. Examine the data that suggests insulin sensitivity may be enhanced by intermittent fasting, providing women in their 60s and older with a possible defence against age-related metabolic diseases.

- **Mental Health and Consistency of Mood**

A satisfying existence is essential to mental and emotional health. Discover the psychological advantages of intermittent fasting, such as its possible effects on emotional resilience and mood stability, which may provide women over 60 a more comprehensive approach to overall wellbeing.

- **Maintaining a Sustainable Weight Loss**

Keeping a healthy weight is a persistent issue for many women. Examine how intermittent fasting, which takes into consideration the particular difficulties and objectives faced by women over 60, may provide a durable and customised strategy to weight control.

• Assessing Individual Needs

One guiding thread in the complex fabric of well-being is uniqueness. It is crucial to acknowledge the distinct requirements, inclinations, and situations of every lady beyond the age of sixty before we start the intermittent fasting adventure. This chapter functions as a compass, providing direction on how to evaluate and customise the intermittent fasting strategy to meet specific needs.

1. Assessment of Health Status

Effective intermittent fasting is based on an awareness of one's present state of health. Examine the significance of doing a comprehensive health evaluation, which should include speaking with medical experts, in order to detect any dietary inadequacies, pre-existing diseases, or contraindications that could affect the fasting experience.

2. Individual Lifestyle Factors

Each woman over sixty adds her own unique set of lifestyle variables to the mix. Analyse how stress levels, sleep habits, work schedules, and daily routines affect the viability and effectiveness of intermittent fasting. Find out how to alter fasting schedules and tactics to suit personal preferences.

3. Dietary Restrictions and Preferences

Dietary decisions and intermittent fasting interact in a complex and highly personalised way. Look at ways to work around dietary restrictions, such as vegetarianism or a particular food allergy, to make sure the fasting strategy you choose still meets your requirements nutritionally and has the intended health effects.

4. Creating Practical Objectives

Setting attainable and unambiguous objectives is essential to the success of any health programme. This section helps women over 60 create individualised, achievable objectives for intermittent fasting that take into account things like energy levels, managing weight, and improving general health.

5. Modifying Fasting Schedules

There isn't a single intermittent fasting plan that works for everyone. Discover the several fasting methods, such as eating inside a certain window of time or fasting on alternate days, and discover how to modify them to suit your own requirements. This involves taking into account possible alterations and progressive adjustments depending on the body's input and development.

6. Tracking Development and Modifying

An essential component of successful intermittent fasting is ongoing self-evaluation. Examine methods for keeping track of developments, identifying indications of good adjustment or possible difficulties, and modifying the fasting strategy as necessary. This flexible approach guarantees that the journey of intermittent fasting stays dynamic and sensitive to personal requirements.

7. Intentional Consumption

Eating with mindfulness is a crucial part of determining what each person needs. Examine mindful eating and how it affects your experience with intermittent fasting. Find out how increasing awareness of one's eating patterns, food preferences, and body's hunger signals may improve the overall efficacy and enjoyment of intermittent fasting.

8. Social and Emotional Factors

Social ties and emotions are closely related to wellness. Examine the emotional dimensions of eating by addressing emotional triggers, stress-related habits, and the impact of social contexts. Learn how to modify intermittent fasting tactics to account for social and emotional factors while maintaining a sustainable and balanced approach.

9. Tailoring Windows for Fasting

The idea of "fasting windows" is essential to intermittent fasting, and this section offers suggestions on how to tailor these windows according to personal preferences and circadian cycles. Find out how timing your fasts to correspond with your body's natural energy changes may improve your overall experience and maximise the benefits for women over 60.

10. Chronobiology and Sleep Hygiene

A key component of good health, sleep has a close relationship with the effectiveness of intermittent fasting. Examine the connection between fasting, circadian cycles, and good sleep hygiene. Find out how women navigating their 60s may improve their general well-being and sleep quality by coordinating their fasting cycles with their natural biological rhythms.

11. Customizing Dietary Consumption

Fasting is important, but consuming the right foods during feeding periods is just as important. Look for ways to customise nutrient-dense meals so that women over 60 get the vitamins and minerals they need for their particular health needs and objectives.

12. Establishing a Help Network

An encouraging community may enhance the experience of beginning an intermittent fasting journey. Acquire knowledge about the significance of establishing a support system, including acquaintances, relatives, or virtual groups. Find out how advice, support, and shared experiences may help you stay motivated and succeed over time.

It is clear that intermittent fasting is a flexible and adaptable method rather than a strict prescription as we traverse the complex terrain of evaluating individual requirements. Women over 60 may create a comprehensive intermittent fasting strategy that seamlessly fits with their own path towards well-being by taking into account their health state, lifestyle considerations, emotional well-being, and personalised preferences.

- ## Choosing the Right Fasting Window

Examine the many fasting windows that are often used in intermittent fasting, including alternate-day fasting, 16/8 fasting, and time-restricted eating. To ensure that your choice is well-informed, get familiar with the subtleties of each strategy, including the length of the fasting and feeding times.

1. Chrononutrition and Circadian Rhythms

Explore the science of chrononutrition and circadian rhythms to learn how the body's internal clock affects metabolism. Discover how the efficacy of intermittent fasting may be increased by lining up fasting windows with natural circadian cycles, which may optimize energy levels and metabolic function for women over the age of 60.

2. Daytime vs. Nighttime Fasting

Examine the pros and drawbacks of fasting in the morning and the evening, taking into account how chronotype, daily routines, and personal preferences might affect the window of time during which to fast. Learn about the possible advantages and difficulties of these strategies as well as how to modify them to meet different lifestyles.

3. Personalised Fasting Periods

Since there are differences across fasting windows, this section delves into the art of customization. Discover how to modify the length of a fast to suit your requirements, objectives, and comfort level. Learn how to embrace the adaptability of intermittent fasting, which enables customized modifications as situations change.

4. Strategies for Gradual Adaptation

Making the switch to a new fasting regimen needs careful planning. Discover how to ease women over 60 into the window of time that they have selected for fasting, reducing the likelihood of pain and increasing the likelihood of long-term success. Examine methods for gradually modifying the length and severity of fasting sessions.

5. Harmonising Nutrition Consumption and Fasting

Selecting the ideal fasting window requires striking a careful balance between feeding the body during eating windows and going without food for extended periods. Advice on finding the right balance is given in this section to make sure that women over 60 get the vitamins, minerals, and other vital nutrients they need for long-term health.

Chapter 2

Nourishing the Body

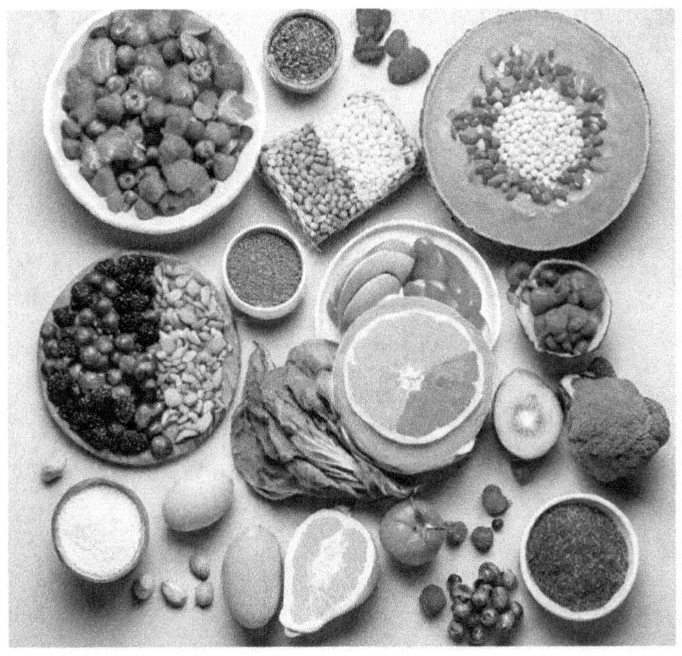

The Importance of Nutrient-Rich Foods

1. Important Elements for Women Over 60

Examine the special dietary requirements for women who are approaching or have reached their sixth decade. Recognize the critical function that certain nutrients play in maintaining general well-being throughout the aging process, from antioxidants for cellular protection to calcium and vitamin D for bone health.

2. Dietary Customisation for Health

This section explores the significance of customizing diets to achieve specific health objectives and treat possible inadequacies, taking into account the fact that nutritional needs vary. Learn how women over 60 who practice intermittent fasting may improve their immune systems, energy levels, and cognitive function by tailoring their nutritional intake.

3. Antioxidant-Rich Foods: Their Power

The unsung heroes of the fight against inflammation and oxidative stress are antioxidants. Examine the origins of foods high in antioxidants and their potential to strengthen cellular health, prevent age-related damage, and lengthen life expectancy.

4. Omega-3 Fatty Acids for Optimal Mental Health

As we age, one of the main concerns is cognitive health, and omega-3 fatty acids become important participants in this field. Explore the origins and advantages of omega-3 fatty acids and how they may support women over 60's mental health, emotional stability, and memory recall.

5. Plant-Based Proteins to Promote Healthy Muscles

Healthy aging depends on maintaining muscular mass and strength. Consider how plant-based proteins may help maintain the health of muscles in women over 60 by offering nutrient-dense, long-lasting choices that suit their dietary needs and intermittent fasting objectives.

6. Micronutrient Balance and Hydration

Staying hydrated is always important, but as we get older, it becomes even more important. Learn how optimal fluid intake enhances nutrient absorption and adds to overall vitality for women over 60 by exploring the link between micronutrient balance and sufficient hydration.

7. High-Fibre Foods to Promote Digestive Health

Foods high in fiber are essential for maintaining digestive health, which is the cornerstone of general well-being. Discover the advantages of including fiber in your diet, which include fostering regular bowel movements, gut health, and the avoidance of digestive problems that are often linked to aging.

Essential Nutrients for Women Over 60

1. Calcium and Vitamin D: Protectors of Healthy Bones

Growing older often raises concerns about bone health, making sufficient calcium and vitamin D consumption essential. Examine how these vital nutrients cooperate to treat common issues like osteoporosis in women over 60, preserve bone density, lower the chance of fractures, and increase overall skeletal strength.

2. Iron: Filling Up Energy Stores

Energy fluctuations may develop in women over 60 due to hormonal changes. Learn about the importance of iron, which is needed to make hemoglobin, the molecule that carries oxygen throughout the blood. Find out how sustaining appropriate amounts of iron might help prevent tiredness and promote continuous energy throughout the day.

3. B Vitamins: Cellular Energy and Cognitive Support

The B-vitamin complex, which includes folate, B6, and B12, shows promise for improving cognitive performance and cellular energy generation. Examine how these nutrients affect the body's energy metabolism, preserve mental clarity, and promote nerve health—all of which are important factors to take into account for women coping with the aging process.

4. Omega-3 Fatty Acids: Promoting the Health of the Brain

When it comes to cognitive vigor, omega-3 fatty acids—EPA and DHA in particular—take center stage. Examine the roles that these important fats play in maintaining brain health, helping with memory retention, slowing down cognitive aging, and maybe even easing some of the emotional difficulties associated with growing older.

5. Antioxidants: Protectors Against Ageing of Cells

Inflammation and oxidative stress are closely related to aging. Examine how antioxidants, including vitamins C and E, work to squelch free radicals and shield cells from harm. Recognize how eating a diet high in antioxidant-rich foods may support cellular health and lessen the impacts of aging.

6. Magnesium: Encouraging Cardiovascular and Muscular Health

As women age, the importance of cardiovascular health and muscle function increases, with magnesium emerging as a critical component. Discover the many uses of magnesium, including blood pressure support, heart rhythm support, muscular function maintenance, and cramp prevention.

7. Fibre: An Enzyme for Digestive Health

The goal of comprehensive health increasingly includes digestive well-being. Explore the significance of dietary fiber and how it maintains gut health, facilitates regular bowel movements, and assists in digestion. Learn how eating more foods high in fiber may help with typical digestive issues that come with becoming older.

Comprehending and giving importance to these vital nutrients enables women over 60 to make knowledgeable food decisions, setting the stage for a well-fed, robust, and prosperous trip during the golden years.

8. Vitamin K: Boosting Heart and Bone Health

The importance of vitamin K for cardiovascular health and bone health puts it in the spotlight despite its frequent undervaluation. Explore the ways that vitamin K promotes bone mineralization, appropriate calcium utilization, and cardiovascular health by assisting with blood clotting regulation.

9. Vitamin A: Aiding the Immune System and Vision

Immune system resiliency and vision are essential elements of well-being. Examine how important vitamin A is for keeping your eyes healthy, especially if you want to avoid age-related macular degeneration. Recognize its importance in strengthening the immune system as well, since this is crucial for preventing infections and promoting immunological function in general.

10. Zinc: Skin Health and Immune Protection

The body's immunological defense systems need to be strengthened as we age. Analyze how zinc promotes wound healing and immune system function. Discover the role that this vital mineral plays in preserving the health of your skin, which is often linked to general well-being and a glowing look.

11. Potassium: Blood Pressure Balancing

The delicate balance of potassium in the body is also a component of cardiovascular health. Examine how this vital mineral helps control blood pressure and may lower the risk of hypertension, which is a common worry for women in their 60s and beyond.

12. Vitamin E: Antioxidant Defence and Skin Vitality

Vitamin E enhances skin vitality and antioxidant defense. Examine how this vitamin helps to preserve the flexibility of the skin, which may help to lessen the signs of aging. Recognize its function as a strong antioxidant as well, protecting the body from oxidative stress and promoting general cellular health.

13. Hydration and Sodium: Electrolyte Equilibrium

Although there is always a warning associated with salt, electrolyte balance is crucial for both hydration and general health. Discover how sodium's delicate balance affects the body's ability to maintain appropriate fluid balance, which is essential for maintaining hydration and several physiological processes.

- **Tailoring Diets for Health**

Personal Health Objectives

This section highlights the need to define individualized goals because health goals vary and are unique. A tailored and efficient nutritional strategy is ensured by customizing the diet to match particular objectives, such as controlling weight, promoting bone health, improving cognitive function, or treating certain medical issues.

Nutritional Preferences and Limitations

Every woman over sixty has her own unique set of dietary requirements and sometimes preferences. It is crucial to recognize and take into account the influences of personal preferences, cultural norms, or medical needs. Look at how modifying diets to fit tastes may improve adherence and pleasure, adding enjoyment and sustainability to the nutritional journey.

Personalised Macronutrient Equilibriums

Dietary customization is significantly influenced by the ratio of macronutrients, including proteins, carbs, and fats. Discuss the need to modify the ratios of macronutrients according to the demands of each person. To preserve muscle, for instance, some women may benefit from consuming more protein, while others may choose to prioritize healthy fats for cardiovascular support.

Getting Used to Changes in Metabolism

Aging-related metabolic alterations impact the body's nutrition utilization and processing. This part examines how crucial it is to modify eating habits to account for these changes in metabolism. Optimizing energy expenditure and metabolic rate to determine nutrition distribution and calorie intake promotes overall metabolic health.

Timing of Nutrients and Strategies for Fasting

The timing of nutritional intake becomes very important for women who fast intermittently. Examine the ways that meals that are customized to coincide with fasting windows might boost metabolic processes, increase energy levels, and improve the overall efficacy of intermittent fasting in women who are over 60.

Taking Care of Inadequate Nutrition

Some dietary deficits may become more common as people age. Discover how addressing certain shortages with diets—like those for calcium, vitamin B12, or D—can reduce health risks and improve wellbeing in general. Adapting nutrient intake through routine health evaluations guarantees a proactive and preventative strategy.

Harmonising Satisfying and Nutrient-Dense Foods

Eating should not be sacrificed to meet nutritional objectives. Learn how to balance meals that are high in nutrients with those that are satisfying and enjoyable. A good and long-lasting connection with food is encouraged by designing diets that provide a range of flavors and sensations in addition to physical wellness.

Intermittent Fasting-friendly Ingredients

- **Components that are suitable for intermittent fasting**

To optimize the health advantages of fasting and promote general well-being, starting an intermittent fasting journey requires thoughtful item selection in addition to meal scheduling. This chapter delves into a wide range of substances that are suitable for intermittent fasting, offering a diverse range of choices that complement the objectives of women over 60 who engage in this technique.

- **Proteins That Are Lean for Extended Energy**

To keep energy levels up and muscle mass intact during fasting periods, lean protein intake is an absolute need. Look at choices like fish, chicken, tofu, lean meat, and lentils. While promoting feelings of fullness, these protein sources provide the necessary amino acids.

- **Plants High in Fibre for a Healthy Digestive System**

Vegetables that are high in fiber are the foundation of a balanced diet. Broccoli, cauliflower, Brussels sprouts, carrots, and leafy greens all support digestive health while offering vital nutrients. A sense of fullness is enhanced by these substances, which helps people fast more effectively.

- **Mind and Body Benefits from Good Fats**

For mental clarity and fullness, include healthy fats in your diet. Rich foods high in omega-3 fatty acids include avocados, nuts, seeds, olive oil, and fatty seafood. Women over 60 may better control their appetite during fasting times thanks to these fats, which help promote brain function and a feeling of fullness.

- **Whole Grains for Long-Term Energy Output**

When it comes to giving off energy gradually, whole grains are beneficial. Nutrient-dense foods that include complex carbs, fiber, and important vitamins include quinoa, brown rice, oats, and barley. Throughout the day, these components provide sustained energy and blood sugar stabilization.

- **Naturally Sweet Fruits with Low Glycemic**

Including low-glycemic fruits in meals brings sweetness naturally and doesn't put blood sugar levels over the roof. While minimizing the influence on insulin response during times of fasting, berries, apples, pears, and citrus fruits are good sources of fiber, vitamins, and antioxidants.

- ## The Calcium Content of Dairy and Dairy Alternatives

Maintaining optimal bone health requires consuming enough calcium. One way to meet your calcium needs is by consuming low-fat dairy products or fortified dairy substitutes like soy or almond milk. Women over 60 may keep strong, robust bones with the help of these nutrients.

- ## Add Flavour Without Calories Using Herbs and Spices

For increasing flavor without gaining additional calories, herbs and spices are helpful. Add flavors to your food by adding things like cilantro, basil, ginger, garlic, and turmeric. Apart from adding diversity to the food, these additives may also have health advantages.

- ## Teas made with herbs and water to stay hydrated

When fasting, staying hydrated is essential. For remaining hydrated without breaking the fast, water, herbal teas, and water flavored with fruits or herbs are great options. Drinking enough water facilitates digestion, boosts energy levels, and controls appetite.

- **Gut Health Benefits of Fermented Foods**

Healthy probiotics are introduced to the gut via fermented foods such as kimchi, kefir, sauerkraut, and yogurt. Especially while fasting intermittently, it is critical to have a healthy gut microbiota for proper digestion and general health.

- **Filling and Rich in Nutrient Broths**

Rich in nutrients broths may be a filling and healthy source of minerals during fasting times. For added hydration, critical nutrients, and appetite management, choose miso soup, vegetable broth, or bone broth.

These varied and nutrient-dense items allow women over 60 to create a tasty, well-balanced intermittent fasting meal that supports them throughout their eating windows and helps them reach their health objectives.

Powerhouse Foods for Energy

1. Oats:
Long-Term Energy Release

Oats are rich in fiber and complex carbs, making them a nutritious powerhouse. They assist in maintaining stable blood sugar levels during fasting times by releasing energy gradually and steadily. B vitamins, which are also included in oats, are essential for energy metabolism.

2. Natural Electrolytes and Carbohydrates in Bananas

Packed with natural sugars, potassium, and vitamin B6, bananas are nature's energy bars. Their carbohydrate and electrolyte content makes them a perfect snack for sustaining muscular function and refueling throughout mealtimes.

3 Quinoa:
Full of Nutrients and Protein

Being a complete protein source that includes all of the necessary amino acids, quinoa stands apart. In addition to complex carbs, fiber, iron, and magnesium, this ancient grain also contributes to general nutritional support and prolonged energy.

1. **Salmon:**
   The Benefits of Omega-3 Fatty Acids to the Brain

Omega-3 fatty acids, especially EPA and DHA, which are abundant in salmon, promote cognitive performance and brain health. These heart-healthy fats provide a sustained energy supply and support a healthy cardiovascular system.

2. **Almonds:**
   Protein and Good Fats

Almonds are a nutrient-dense powerhouse that combines fiber, protein, and healthy fats. Almonds' monounsaturated fats provide you with long-lasting energy, and their high protein content helps you maintain muscle during intermittent fasting.

3. **Sweet Potatoes:**
   Nutrients and Complex Carbohydrates

Sweet potatoes are a great source of fiber, complex carbs, and important minerals like potassium and vitamin A. Because they release energy gradually due to their delayed digestion, they are the perfect fuel for prolonged use.

4. Probiotics and Protein in Greek Yoghurt

A high-protein choice that also adds good probiotics for intestinal health is Greek yogurt. Maintaining muscle mass requires protein, and probiotics help maintain intestinal health, which boosts general energy and vigor.

5. Micronutrients and Iron in Dark Leafy Greens

Dark leafy vegetables, including kale and spinach, are high in vitamins and iron. For the body to produce energy and transfer oxygen, iron is essential. Including these greens guarantees an increase in nutrients that raise vitality levels all around.

6. Chia Seeds: Fibre and Omega-3s

Chia seeds are rich in protein, fiber, and omega-3 fatty acids, making them a nutritional powerhouse. While fiber promotes digestive health and aids in hunger control, omega-3s assist in maintaining brain function and provide long-lasting energy.

7. Berries: Natural Sugars and Antioxidants

Strawberries, raspberries, and blueberries are just a few of the berries that are rich in natural sugars and antioxidants. The natural sugars provide a rapid energy boost without raising blood sugar levels, while the antioxidants fight oxidative stress.

Chapter 3

Delicious Breakfast Recipes

- ## Berry Bliss Smoothie Bowl

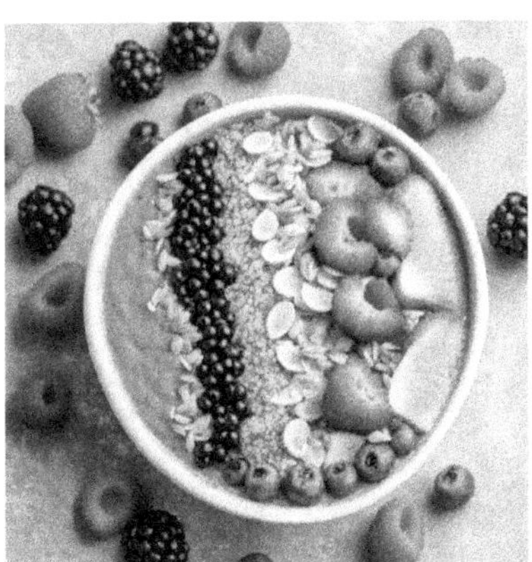

Ingredients:

- One cup of frozen mixed berries, including raspberries, blueberries, and strawberries
- one frozen, sliced, ripe banana
- Half a cup of Greek yogurt
- 1/4 cup of rolled oats
- a single spoonful of chia seeds
- One tsp almond butter

- 1/2 cup almond milk (or any other kind of milk you want)
- One teaspoon of optionally sweetened maple syrup or honey

Toppers: Almond slices, chia seeds, granola, sliced banana, and fresh berries

Guidelines:

1. Set Up the Foundation:

The frozen mixed berries, frozen banana slices, Greek yogurt, rolled oats, chia seeds, almond butter, and almond milk should all be combined in a blender.

2. Mix Until Smooth:

Process the ingredients in a high-speed blender until a thick and creamy consistency is reached. You may adjust the thickness by adding a small amount of additional almond milk if the mixture is too thick.

3. Try and sweeten (if desired):

If you want to add more sweetness to the smoothie mixture, taste it and add honey or maple syrup. Blend one more to integrate.

4. Transfer into a bowl:

Make sure the smoothie is thick enough to be spoonable as you pour it into a bowl.

5. Top with Toppings:

Put the toppings in the smoothie bowl's order. For extra texture and nutritional value, top with sliced almonds, granola, fresh berries, banana slices, and more chia seeds.

6. Tailor:

Go ahead and add more of your favorite toppings to your bowl, such as coconut flakes, pumpkin seeds, or a dab of nut butter.

7. Savour right away:

Savor the vibrant flavors and give your day a boost of energy by diving into your berry blast smoothie bowl right now.

- **Green Goddess Power Bowl**

Ingredients:

About the Bowl:

- One cup of chopped, finely kale
- one cup of spinach leaves
- 1/4 cup sliced broccoli florets,
- 1/2 avocado,
- 1/4 cucumber,
- 1/4 cup steamed edamame,
- 1/4 cup cooked quinoa, and
- 1 tablespoon cooked pumpkin seeds
- one spoonful of sunflower seeds

Regarding the Dressed Green Goddess:

- one-fourth cup of Greek yogurt, plain
- one-fourth cup of fresh basil leaves
- one-fourth cup of fresh parsley leaves
- one sliced green onion
- One minced garlic clove
- one tablespoon of lemon juice
- Two tsp extra virgin olive oil
- Add salt and pepper to taste.

Guidelines:

Get the Bowl Ready:

1. Greens Foundation:

Layer chopped kale and spinach leaves to form a foundation in a big bowl.

Add Place cooked edamame, steamed broccoli florets, cucumber, and sliced avocado on top of the greens.

2. Boost Quinoa:

In the center of the dish, place a mound of cooked quinoa.

3. Above with Seeds:

For extra crunch and nutritional value, sprinkle sunflower and pumpkin seeds over the dish.

The Green Goddess Dressing should be ready.

4. Mix the ingredients:

Greek yogurt, parsley, basil, minced garlic, green onion, lemon juice, and extra virgin olive oil should all be combined in a food processor or blender.

5. Mix Until Smooth:

Blend until the mixture becomes a creamy, smooth dressing. Season with salt and pepper.

Put together the Power Bowl:

6. Dressing Drizzled Over:

Over the contents of the dish, liberally drizzle with the Green Goddess Dressing.

7. Carefully Toss:

To guarantee that the components are evenly coated with dressing, gently toss them.

8. Decorative elements (Optional):

Add more herbs or a slice of lemon as a garnish if you'd like something new.

9. Serve right away:

To highlight the vivid flavors and textures of the Green Goddess Power Bowl, serve it right away.

Savour the goodness packed with nutrients:

With its well-balanced combination of greens, veggies, protein-rich quinoa, and a tasty dressing, this Green Goddess Power Bowl is a nutrient-dense joy. This power bowl is full of vitamins, minerals, and antioxidants that will not only satisfy your palate but also provide your body with the nutrients and energy it needs.

Satisfying Breakfast Soups

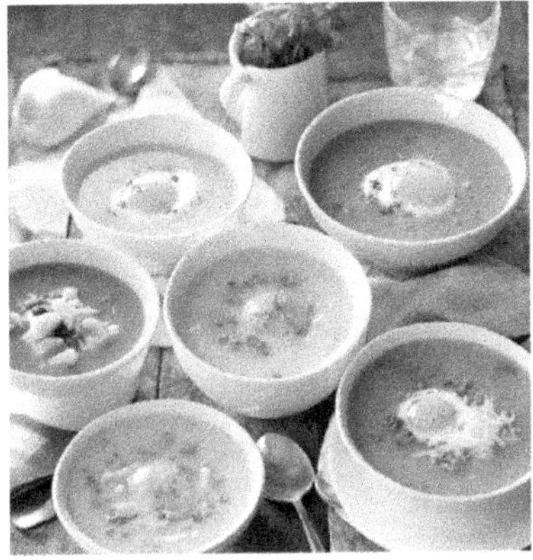

- **Golden Turmeric Broth**

Ingredients:

- cups of homemade or store-bought vegetable broth
- one tablespoon of powdered turmeric
- One tsp finely grated ginger
- minced two garlic cloves
- Half an onion, chopped; one medium carrot; one celery stalk;
- One cup of finely chopped kale
- Half a cup of coconut milk
- One tsp extra virgin olive oil
- Add salt and pepper to taste.
- Use fresh parsley or cilantro as a garnish (optional).
- A freshly squeezed lemon juice (optional)

Guidelines:

1. Aromatics sautéed:

Olive oil should be warmed over medium heat in a large saucepan. Add the minced garlic, chopped onions, and grated ginger. Onions should be sautéed until fragrant and transparent.

2. Include some turmeric:

Infuse the aromatics and oil with the turmeric powder by stirring it in. The broth's color and flavor are improved by this stage.

3. Compostables In:

Toss in the chopped kale, celery, and carrot slices. Toss to coat the veggies with the oil flavored with turmeric and sauté briefly.

4. Fill with Broth:

After adding the vegetable broth, slowly bring the mixture to a boil. Once the veggies are soft, lower the heat to a simmer and continue cooking them.

5. Mix with Coconut Milk:

To get a creamy, golden broth, carefully mix in the coconut milk after adding it. Give the flavors five to seven minutes on low heat to mingle.

6. To Taste, Season:

To taste, add more salt and pepper to the broth. Taste and adjust the seasoning.

7. Serve Warm:

Pour the Golden Turmeric Broth into bowls, making sure that each portion has a good mixture of veggies.

8. Arrange and Savour:

For a pop of freshness, add some parsley or cilantro as a garnish. Optionally, just before serving, pour a little fresh lemon juice into each dish.

9. Go in pairs or have a solo drink:

You may have the Golden Turmeric Broth by itself as a soothing beverage or combine it with your preferred grains, noodles, or protein to make a more substantial meal.

10. Taste the Heat:

Enjoy the warmth and nutrition of this fragrant and tasty Golden Turmeric Broth by taking a sip.

Note: Depending on your tastes and what you have in your kitchen, feel free to change the recipe by adding different veggies like bell peppers, mushrooms, or spinach.

- **Vegetable Medley Morning Soup**

Ingredients list:

- A single spoonful of olive oil
- 1 small onion, diced finely
- One chopped carrot, one diced celery stalk, one diced bell pepper (any color), one diced zucchini, one cup of chopped cherry tomatoes, and two minced garlic cloves
- Four cups of broth made with vegetables
- One tsp. of dried thyme
- One tsp. of dried oregano
- Add salt and pepper to taste.
- Two cups chopped spinach or kale
- 1 cup of brown rice or cooked quinoa (optional)
- For garnish, use fresh herbs like parsley or chives.
- Serve with slices of lemon, if desired.

Guidelines:

1. Aromatics sautéed:

Olive oil should be heated over medium heat in a large saucepan. Add the chopped onions and garlic, and sauté until the onions become translucent and aromatic.

2. Include Vegetables:

To the saucepan, add the chopped carrots, celery, bell pepper, zucchini, and cherry tomatoes. Let the veggies soften for a few minutes while they are sautéing.

3. Fill with Broth:

Make sure the veggies are covered when you pour in the vegetable broth. Heat the mixture until it gently boils.

4. Use herbs to season:

Add salt, pepper, dried oregano, and dried thyme. Depending on your own tastes, adjust the seasoning.

5. Simmer

For around 15 to 20 minutes, lower the heat to a simmer and let the soup stew, enabling the flavors to combine and the veggies to soften.

6. Include Leafy Greens:

Toss in with chopped kale or spinach just before serving. Stir until wilted, adding more greens.

7. Grains Not Required:

Cooked quinoa or brown rice may be added to the soup pot for a heartier flavor. Let it warm through after giving it a good stir.

8. Add a garnish and serve:

The Vegetable Medley Morning Soup should be ladled into bowls. Use fresh herbs like chives or parsley as a garnish.

9. Optionally, add a zesty kick:

To add a zesty touch, serve the soup with slices of lemon. Fresh lemon juice should be squeezed into your dish just before eating.

10. Savor a Filling Breakfast:

This Vegetable Medley Morning Soup is a healthy and nourishing way to start the day. Savour its warmth and sustenance.

A lovely blend of vibrant veggies, fragrant herbs, and optional grains for the extra body is found in this soup. For a cool breakfast treat, feel free to modify the recipe using your preferred veggies or according to what's in season.

Chapter 4

Wholesome Lunch Creations

- ## Mediterranean Chickpea Salad

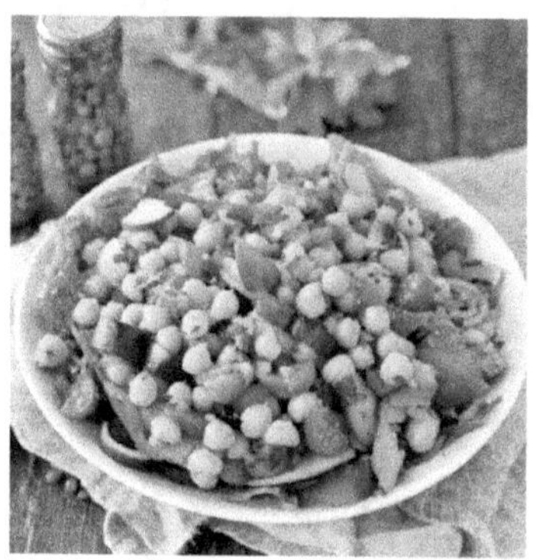

Ingredients:

- combine 2 cans (15 ounces each) of chickpeas,
- 1 cucumber, diced, drained, and rinsed, diced,
- a cup of cherry tomatoes,
- halved red bell pepper, diced yellow bell pepper, diced
- 1/2 red onion, finely chopped,
- 1/2 cup Kalamata olives, sliced,

- 1/2 cup feta cheese, crumbled,
- 1/4 cup fresh parsley, chopped,
- 1/4 cup fresh mint.

For the dressing,

- A quarter cup of extra virgin olive oil
- Two teaspoons of vinegar made from red wine
- One tsp Dijon mustard
- One minced garlic clove
- One tsp. of dried oregano
- Add salt and black pepper to taste.

Guidelines:

1. Get the chickpeas ready.

The rinsed and drained chickpeas should be combined in a big basin.

2. Cut Up Vegetables:

Cut the cherry tomatoes, red and yellow bell peppers, cucumber, and red onion into small pieces. Place them in the basin with the chickpeas.

3. Put Feta and Olives in:

Separate the feta cheese and cut the Kalamata olives. Combine them with the other veggies in the dish.

4. Fresh Plants:

To add a burst of freshness to the salad, chop some fresh mint and parsley.

5. Whisk the Dressing:

Minced garlic, dried oregano, Dijon mustard, red wine vinegar, extra virgin olive oil, salt, and black pepper should all be combined in a small bowl. Stir in the salt to taste.

6. Mix the salad with the dressing.

Drizzle the chickpea and veggie mixture with the dressing. Mix everything gently until well mixed and the dressing is distributed evenly.

7. Relax and season:

To enable the flavors to marinade, cover the salad dish and place it in the refrigerator for at least half an hour.

8. Proceed to serve and relish:

Toss the salad one last time and serve cold. Add a sprinkling of feta cheese or more fresh herbs as an optional garnish.

Optional Pairings:

For a light and filling lunch, try the Mediterranean Chickpea Salad on its own. You can also serve it as a side dish for your next get-together or with grilled chicken or fish.

- **Citrus Walnut Kale Salad**

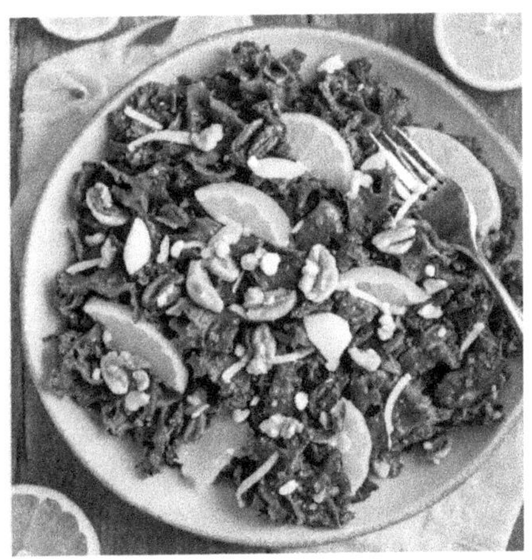

Ingredients:

- 1 bunch kale, stems removed and finely cut leaves
- 1 cup fresh or canned mandarin orange segments
- 1/2 cup toasted chopped walnuts
- Optional: 1/4 cup crumbled feta cheese

- 1/4 cup pomegranate arils or dried cranberries
- 1/4 cup finely sliced red onion
- One orange's zest

To make the dressing:

- 3 tbsp extra virgin olive oil
- 2 tbsp. fresh orange juice
- 1 tbsp honey (or maple syrup)
- 1 tbsp. Dijon mustard
- To taste, add salt and black pepper for seasoning.

Instructions:

1. Prepare the Kale:

Remove the kale leaves' stems and finely slice the leaves. In a large salad dish, place the sliced kale.

2. Toast the walnuts:

Toast the chopped walnuts in a dry pan over medium heat until aromatic and lightly toasted. To avoid scorching, stir often. Take off the heat source and let it cool.

3. Salad Assemble:

Toss the sliced kale with the mandarin orange segments, toasted walnuts, dried cranberries or pomegranate arils, and sliced red onion.

4. Prepare the Dressing:

Whisk together extra-virgin olive oil, fresh orange juice, honey or maple syrup, and Dijon mustard, and season with salt and black pepper in a small bowl.

5. Salad dressing:

Drizzle the salad dressing over the items. Massage the kale leaves for a minute or two with clean hands. Massaging the kale softens it and enables the flavors to combine.

6. Add the zest of an orange:

Sprinkle the salad with the zest of one orange. The citrus zest gives a burst of flavor and freshness to the dish.

7. Feta Topping (Optional):

Crumble feta cheese over the salad if preferred for a creamy and tangy flavour. This is optional and may be left out if you want a dairy-free version.

8. Toss the coin once more:

Toss the salad one more time to ensure that all of the components are well-coated with the dressing.

9. Optional chilling:

To enable the flavors to meld, chill the salad in the refrigerator for 15-30 minutes before serving.

10. Serve and have fun:

Serve the Citrus Walnut Kale Salad separately or as a side dish. It's a colorful and nutrient-dense salad that combines the benefits of citrus, crisp walnuts, and robust kale.

- **Lentil and Vegetable Stew**

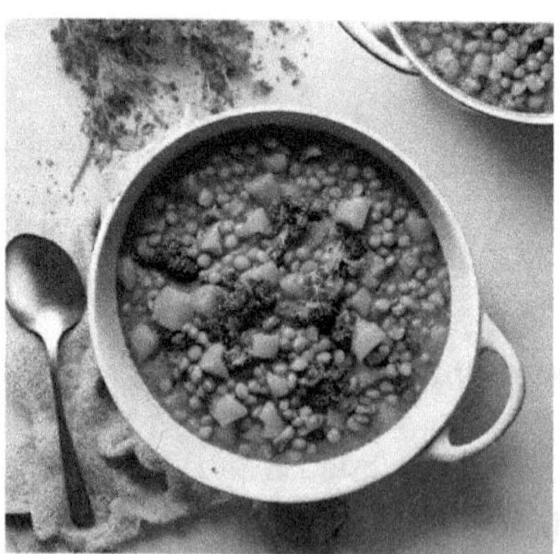

Ingredients:

- 1 cup washed and drained dried lentils, either brown or green
- One big onion, chopped
- minced three garlic cloves
- Two carrots, chopped and peeled
- two celery stalks, chopped
- One chopped bell pepper of any hue
- one chopped zucchini
- One can, weighing fourteen ounces of sliced tomatoes
- 1 teaspoon of ground cumin and 4 cups of vegetable broth
- one tsp finely ground coriander
- A single tsp of smoky paprika
- half a teaspoon of powdered turmeric
- one bay leaf
- Add salt and black pepper to taste.
- Two teaspoons of olive oil
- Garnish with fresh parsley, if desired.
- Serve with slices of lemon, if desired.

Guidelines:

1. **Aromatics sautéed:**

Olive oil should be warmed over medium heat in a large saucepan. Add the chopped onions and garlic, and cook until the onions start to become aromatic and transparent.

2. Incorporate Spices and Lentils:

Rinse the lentils and add them to the pot along with the smoked paprika, turmeric powder, powdered cumin, ground coriander, salt, and black pepper. Coat the lentils with the fragrant spices by stirring.

3. Compostables In:

Add the bell pepper, zucchini, celery, and chopped carrots to the saucepan. Let the veggies soften for a few minutes while they are sautéing.

4. Broth with Tomatoes:

Add the veggie broth and diced tomatoes (with juice) from the can. Toss to mix well.

5. Modify and Reduce:

When necessary, adjust the seasoning and add the bay leaf. Once the stew reaches a soft boil, lower the heat so that it simmers. After the lentils and veggies are soft, simmer the mixture covered for 25 to 30 minutes.

6. Verify Coherence:

You may adjust the consistency of the stew by adding more vegetable broth if it appears too thick.

Modify the Seasoning:

Before serving, check the seasoning by tasting. If needed, add more salt, pepper, or spices.

7. Serve Warm:

Fill dishes with the Lentil and Vegetable Stew. Garnish with parsley, if preferred.

8. Optional: Lemon Wedges

Accompany the stew with slices of lemon. Fresh lemon juice gives a delightfully zesty boost to the stew when squeezed over it just before serving.

9. Savour the Thick Stew:

Savour this hearty stew made with lentils and vegetables for a filling and healthy dinner. On cold days, it's ideal for staying warm.

- ## Quinoa Minestrone

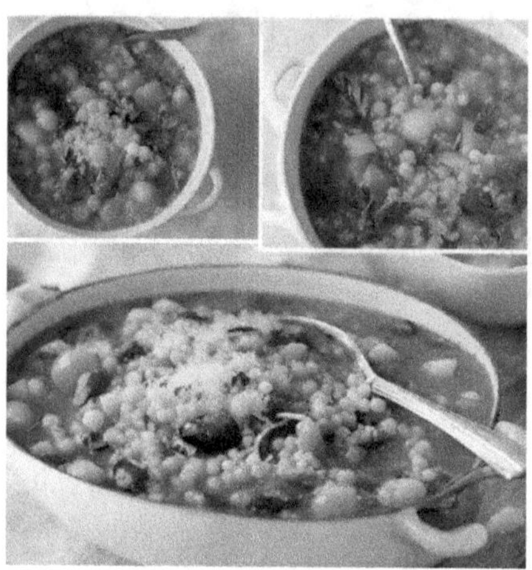

Ingredients:

- Rinse and drain 1 cup of quinoa
- Two teaspoons of olive oil
- One big onion, chopped
- Three chopped garlic cloves, two chopped carrots, two diced celery stalks, one sliced zucchini and one diced can (14 ounces) sliced tomatoes
- Cannellini beans, one (15-ounce can), drained and rinsed
- One teaspoon of dried oregano and four cups of vegetable broth
- one tsp of dried basil
- Half a teaspoon of thyme, dry

- Add salt and black pepper to taste.
- Chopped two cups of spinach or greens
- 1/2 cup elbow or ditalini-style tiny pasta
- Grated Parmesan cheese (optional) to be served
- Garnish with fresh basil, if desired.

Guidelines:

Clean Quinoa:

Wash the quinoa in cold water and reserve.

Aromatics sautéed:

Olive oil should be warmed over medium heat in a large saucepan. Add the chopped onions and garlic, and cook until the onions become fragrant and transparent.

Include Vegetables:

To the saucepan, add the chopped carrots, celery, and zucchini. Let the veggies soften for a few minutes while they are sautéing.

Broth with Tomatoes:

Add the cannellini beans, vegetable broth, and chopped tomatoes with juice. Toss to mix well.

Seasoning /

Stir in the dried thyme, dried basil, dried oregano, black pepper, and salt. To suit your taste, adjust the seasoning.

Heat to a boil:

Once the soup reaches a soft boil, lower the heat and let it simmer. To allow the flavors to mingle, cover and simmer for around fifteen minutes.

Put Pasta and Quinoa Here:

Place a little spaghetti in the saucepan with the washed quinoa. Simmer the pasta and quinoa for a further 10 to 15 minutes, or until they are done.

Add the greens and stir:

Add chopped spinach or kale to the soup, stirring to allow it to wilt.

Verify Coherence:

You may adjust the soup's consistency by adding more vegetable broth if it's too thick.

Serve Warm:

Divide the Quinoa Minestrone evenly among bowls. Garnish each dish with freshly chopped basil and grated Parmesan cheese, if desired, to enhance the flavor.

Savour a Balanced Lunch:

Warm up this filling and healthy Quinoa Minestrone and enjoy the flavorful blend of quinoa, veggies, and fragrant herbs.

This Quinoa Minestrone is a hearty, high-protein take on the traditional Italian soup. This hearty and filling dish is ideal for every day of the week since it's loaded with quinoa, veggies, and delicious herbs.

Chapter 5

Delectable Dinner Delights

- **Balanced One-Pan Meals**

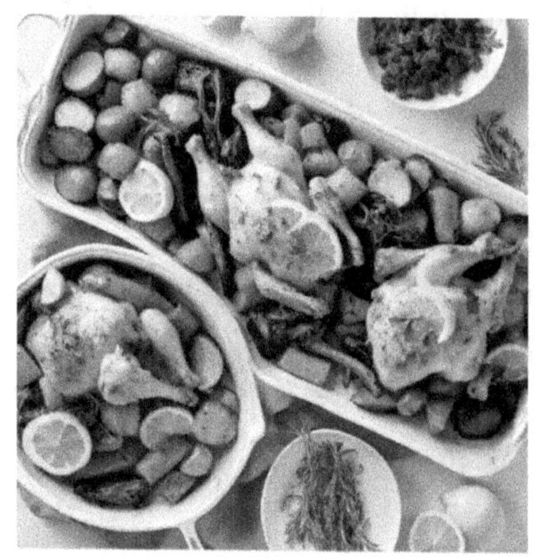

Roasted Vegetables and Lemon Herb Chicken

Ingredients:

- skin- and bone-free chicken breasts
- Half a pound of baby potatoes
- One cup of tiny carrots
- broccoli florets in one cup
- Two teaspoons of olive oil

- Three chopped garlic cloves and one sliced lemon
- One tsp. of dried thyme
- one teaspoon of dried rosemary
- Add salt and black pepper to taste.
- For garnish, use fresh parsley.

Guidelines:

1. Warm the oven up to 400°F, or 200°C.

2. Combine olive oil, minced garlic, salt, black pepper, dried thyme, and dried rosemary in a bowl.

3. Coat half of the herb mixture over the chicken breasts before placing them on one side of a large baking sheet.

4. Add the remaining herb combination to the potatoes, carrots, and broccoli and toss. Put them in order on the other side of the baking sheet.

5. Arrange slices of lemon over the meat.

6. Bake for twenty-five to thirty minutes, or until the veggies are soft and the chicken is well cooked.

7. Before serving, sprinkle some fresh parsley on top.

Quinoa and Shrimp Paella

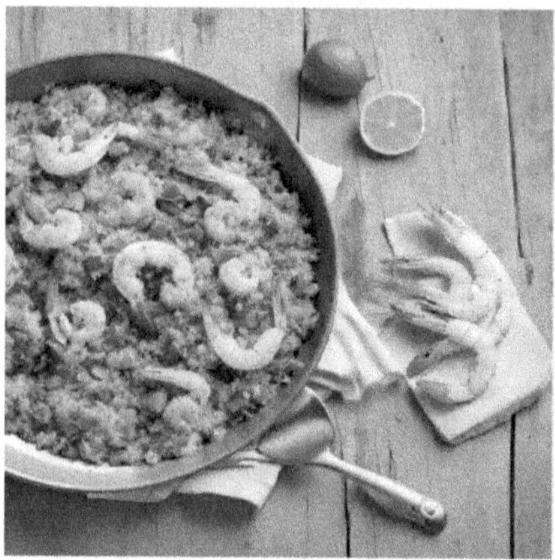

Ingredients:

- Rinse and drain 1 cup of quinoa
- One big prawn pound, deveined and skinned
- One finely sliced onion
- Dice one bell pepper and two tomatoes
- minced three garlic cloves
- Two teaspoons of paprika with smoke
- One teaspoon of finely ground turmeric
- Saffron threads, 1/2 teaspoon (optional)
- One cup of frozen peas and two cups of chicken or veggie broth
- Two teaspoons of olive oil
- Add salt and black pepper to taste.
- Slices of lemon to serve

Guidelines:

1. Olive oil should be heated over medium heat in a big skillet or paella pan.
2. Bell pepper and diced onion should be sautéed till tender.
3. Add the ground turmeric, smoked paprika, chopped garlic, and saffron, if using. Mix well to blend.
4. Stir the quinoa for a minute or two to toast it.
5. After adding the broth, simmer. Cook the quinoa for about 15 minutes, or until it is nearly done.
6. Over the quinoa, arrange the chopped tomatoes, frozen peas, and shrimp. season with salt and pepper.
7. Once the prawns are cooked through and pink, cover and simmer for a further 10 minutes.

Salmon Baked with Veggie Packing and Couscous

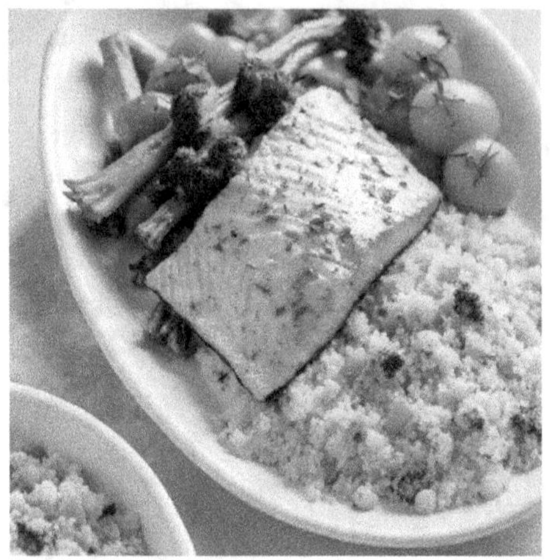

Ingredients:

- four fillets of salmon
- 1-cup cooked couscous
- One cup of cherry tomatoes, cut in half; one zucchini, chopped; one yellow squash, chopped
- One red onion cut thinly
- Two teaspoons of olive oil
- Balsamic vinegar, two teaspoons
- 1 teaspoon of dried Italian herbs
- Add salt and black pepper to taste.
- To garnish, use fresh basil.

Guidelines:

1. Set the oven temperature to 375°F, or 190°C.

2. Combine the dried Italian herbs, olive oil, balsamic vinegar, salt, and black pepper in a bowl.
3. On a large baking sheet, place the salmon fillets in the center.
4. Combine red onion, cherry tomatoes, yellow squash, and zucchini with the olive oil mixture. Stack them on top of the salmon.
5. Bake the salmon for 20 to 25 minutes, or until it's well done and the veggies are soft.
6. Arrange a bed of prepared couscous to accompany the baked salmon. Add fresh basil as a garnish.

Indulgent Desserts with a Healthy Twist

These decadent, guilt-free sweets will satisfy your sweet taste without letting up your resolve to live a better lifestyle.

1. Mousse with avocado and dark chocolate

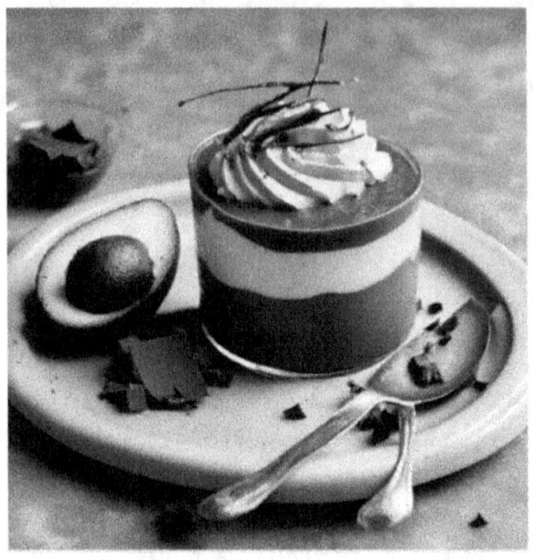

Ingredients:

- Two mature avocados
- Half a cup of cocoa powder, unsweetened
- 1/2 cup unadulterated honey or maple syrup
- one tsp vanilla essence
- a little amount of salt
- To garnish, fresh berries

Guidelines:

1. In a food processor, blend avocados, cocoa powder, vanilla extract, maple syrup or honey, and a little amount of salt until smooth.
2. Transfer the mousse into serving glasses using a spoon, then chill for a minimum of half an hour.

3. Before serving, scatter some fresh berries on top.

2. Panna Cotta with Greek Yoghurt and Honey

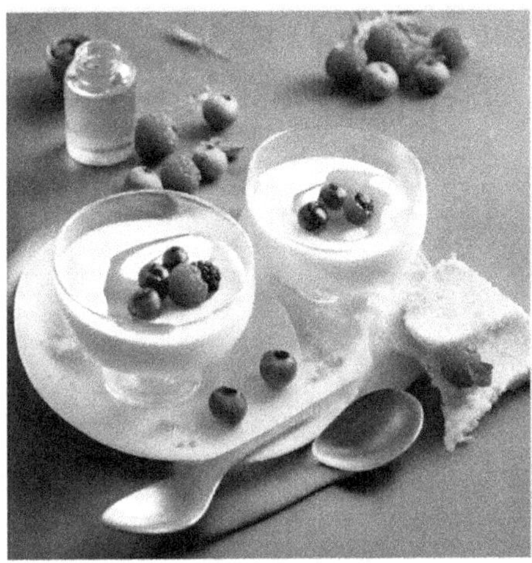

Ingredients:

- Two cups of Greek yogurt, plain
- Half a cup of honey
- Two teaspoons of gelatin and a teaspoon of vanilla extract
- 1/4 cup hot water
- Berries mixed to garnish

Guidelines:

1. Greek yogurt, honey, and vanilla essence should all be well mixed in a bowl.
2. Dissolve the gelatin in warm water in a separate small basin.
3. Blend the yogurt mixture with the gelatin mixture until it's smooth.
4. After pouring the liquid into ramekins, chill them for at least four hours, or until they solidify.
5. To serve, sprinkle some mixed berries on top.

4. Apple Chips with Baked Cinnamon

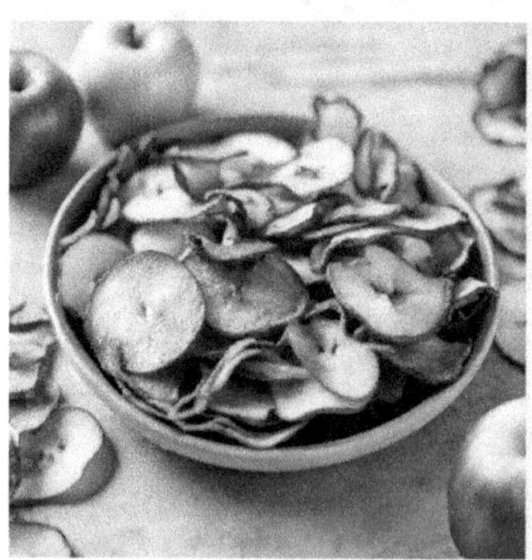

Ingredients:

- Four apples, cut thinly
- one spoonful of cinnamon

- One tablespoon of coconut sugar, if desired

Guidelines:

1. Set oven temperature to 225°F, or 110°C.
2. Toss the apple slices in coconut sugar and cinnamon.
3. Layer the slices one at a time on a baking sheet covered with paper.
4. Bake, rotating the chips halfway through, for 2 to 3 hours, or until they are crisp.
5. Before serving, let them cool.

4. Dessert with Chia Seed Chocolate

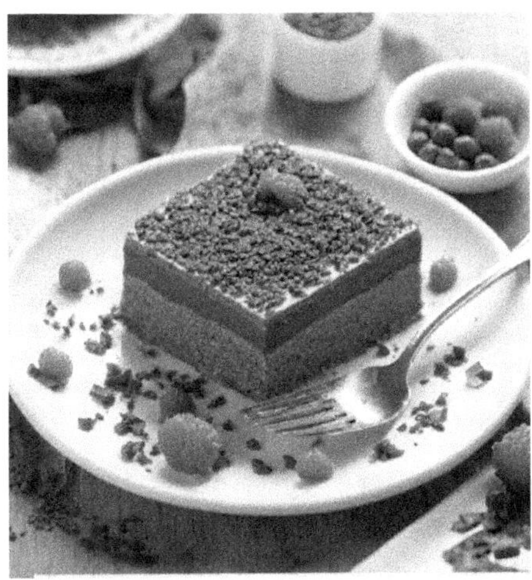

Ingredients:

- one-fourth cup of chia seeds

- One cup of almond milk (or any other kind of milk)
- Two tsp of chocolate powder without sweetness
- Two teaspoons of pure maple syrup
- One-half tsp vanilla extract
- strawberries are cut into slices to serve as a topping

Guidelines:

- Chia seeds, almond milk, vanilla extract, chocolate powder, and maple syrup should all be combined in a bowl.
- Stirring periodically, chill for a minimum of three hours, or overnight.
- When ready to serve, spoon custard into glasses, then top with cut strawberries.

6. Banana Oatmeal Cookies

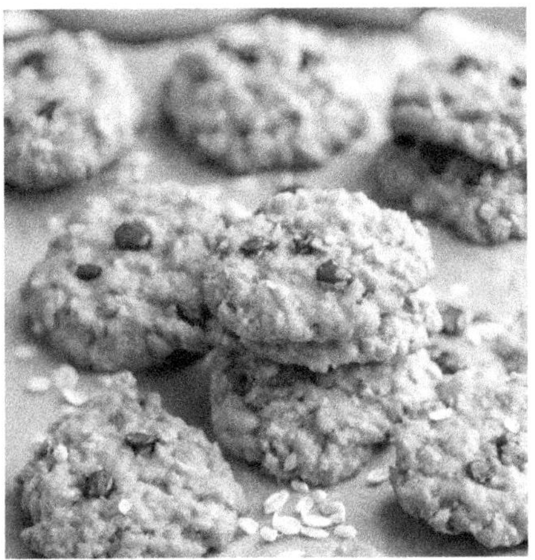

Ingredients:

- two mashed, ripe bananas
- one cup of rolled oats
- One-fourth cup of almond butter
- one-fourth cup of chips made with dark chocolate
- One-half tsp vanilla extract
- a little amount of salt

Guidelines:

1. Turn the oven on to 350°F, or 180°C.
2. Beat together mashed bananas, almond butter, dark chocolate chips, vanilla extract, and a little amount of salt in a bowl.
3. Spoon the mixture onto a baking sheet in spoonfuls.
4. Bake until the edges are golden brown.

5. When ready to eat, let the cookies cool.

You can indulge your sweet tooth while still making healthy choices by trying these desserts, which provide a great balance between pleasure and health. As part of a healthy lifestyle, savor these guilt-free delights.Conclusion: Savoring the Journey to Health and Longevity.

Conclusion:

Savoring the Journey to Health and Longevity

We've covered healthy habits and thoughtful decisions for a happier, healthier life, but it's important to recognize that getting there takes time. Adopting a health-conscious lifestyle does not have to entail giving up the enjoyment of delectable meals and sweets. Rather, it's about choosing with purpose what feeds the body and the spirit.

We have examined the science of fasting, the advantages of fasting for women over 60, the importance of nutrient-rich meals, and how to customize diets for specific requirements via the chapters of this book. We've created a variety of well-balanced one-pan dinners and decadent desserts with a healthy twist to illustrate that eating well can be tasty and interesting.

Remember that developing a healthy connection with food is more important than severe restriction as you set out on your path to life and health. It's about choosing a way of living that enhances your general well-being and makes you happy. Every decision you make, whether it's to enjoy a guilt-free Dark Chocolate Avocado Mousse, a Quinoa Minestrone, or a Golden Turmeric Broth, helps you become a healthier version of yourself.

Every deliberate choice, wholesome meal, and self-care session you make during your health journey adds up to a colorful and robust image of well-being. So enjoy the food, savor the flavors, and commemorate your path towards long life and health. May every step you take be a joyful, purposeful move in the direction of a better, happier self.

THANK YOU FOR CHOOSING US.

We Appreciate Your Kind Support And We Hope You Got Something Out Of It.

If You Enjoy This Book, It Will Be Great To Leave a Review On Amazon . It Means a Lot To Us.